Fix Plantar Fasciitis

S A BURLEY

Fix Plantar Fasciitis

Medical Disclaimer

Before you start any of the exercises or follow any of the recommendations in Fix Plantar Fasciitis it is imperative that you visit your doctor and make sure that you are diagnosed as having Plantar Fasciitis.

You should also consult your doctor at any stage during your recovery before you do anything recommended in Fix Plantar Fasciitis or on the Fix Plantar Fasciitis website.

We do not and cannot accept any liability for any injury or negative effect, or loss, you may encounter by using the information in this book, whether it be physical, mental, financial, or other.

Please see the full terms and conditions on our website FixPlantarFasciitis.com and at the end of this book.

Contents

Introduction

My Painful Plantar Fasciitis Story Could Be Your Easy Plantar Fasciitis Fix

I have experienced Plantar Fasciitis for over twenty years, maybe even longer as I remember having similar pain when I was a child, but then I would get over it quickly.

As an adult at first it started pretty minor and would repeat once every one to two years and last for only between one to three weeks.

Over the years the time between episodes shortened and the pain became gradually worse. However, it was still bearable, so I followed the advice of my doctor, took painkillers, read some information leaflets, did some stretches and thought I must have been doing the 'right' thing because eventually it would start to go away.

But it was never fully going away and about five years ago it suddenly became excruciating and unbearable.

I couldn't see what trigger had brought about the terrible episode, so I went again to my doctor. This time his recommendation was to take pain killers for two weeks and it should go away. Of course, it did not. I asked if there was anything else I could do, and the recommendations were to wear arch supporting shoes, possibly get custom arch supports made (which is a route some friends of mine went down at a high cost and it did not fix their Plantar Fasciitis), and keep taking the pills!

Being barely mobile because of the pain, and being woken up and kept awake at night, I had to take matters into my own hands to see if I could get rid of this thing. I had already done a lot of research over the years into how to fix Plantar Fasciitis, but it was clear that I needed to research all the latest information I could find.

As I'm sure you know if you've ever had it, persistent pain can change every aspect of your life, including creating mental health problems, creating problems with family and friends because of your mood and your lack of physical ability to go places with them, negatively impact your working life and even stop you working in some professions, and is physically and mentally absolutely exhausting.

So, determined to get over Plantar Fasciitis, I read, researched, watched, joined Facebook Groups, and discussed as much Plantar Fasciitis information as I could.

You will find, like me, that the vast amount of the Plantar Fasciitis information available in the world today can be confusing and can very often be contradictory.

You will also find that most of the websites and books about Plantar Fasciitis are brimming with so much information that it takes a massive amount of time to read through it all.

This can be so frustrating, and confusing, when all you really want to do is get better as easily and quickly as possible.

Because of the amount of information to look through in the world today it can become overwhelming and can delay your recovery even more.

I tried everything which was recommended until I could be sure that I knew the things which worked the best for me.

At the same time, I wanted to compile and keep an easy and effective plan in case Plantar Fasciitis ever decided to come back, and ideally I wanted information which would help me to prevent it coming back at all.

Thankfully, I am now Plantar Fasciitis free and have been for a long time. Once, when I slipped into being lazy and not following my own plan, it did hint at coming back, but because I had the information in this book to hand, I was able to quickly make it go away within a few days. And now I just remind myself to check my behaviour day to day!

So, after much time, and much suffering, I have this information in a book format to share it with you so that my pain can be to your benefit. So that your suffering is kept at a minimum and so you are better equipped to deal with any episodes which may arise in the future.

I want you to be able to get over Plantar Fasciitis as quickly and easily as possible, because I know from firsthand (or foot!) experience that it can be utter misery.

The Fix Plantar Fasciitis Book

I have written, re-written, and edited so that I can give you the best experience I can.

I've tried my best through the years of research, trial and error, and very painful experiences to make this book:

- Short
- Straight to the point
- Contain no filler or unnecessary information
- Contain no complicated illustrations
- Contain no unnecessary medical or biological information
- Easy for you to follow
- Easy for you to do
- Easy for you to fit into your day
- Save you massive amounts of time
- Save you potentially large amounts of money on unnecessary treatment.
- Save you potentially large amounts of money on devices, rubs, equipment, and many other items which I spent my own money on to test and find the best ones so that you don't have to!
- Significantly reduce the amount of pain you suffer
- Significantly reduce the amount of time you suffer pain
- Help you prevent recurrences of plantar fasciitis
- Help you quickly stop the progression of any recurrences
- Help you quickly reverse any recurrence at the first signs

If you don't follow the prevention recommendations to the letter, then hopefully the information in this book should help you stop any recurrence from becoming excruciating and also to help you to reduce and get rid of any pain again. But I very much suggest that your aim, as much as possible, is to prevent Plantar Fasciitis pain from coming back.

For me the information provides the shortest, most effective guide to the quickest, easiest and least painful recovery from Plantar Fasciitis, and I strongly believe it can do the same for you.

If you carefully follow what I have put in this book in conjunction with advice you get from your own chosen medical professionals at the time then I believe it is very likely to help you.

If this book doesn't help you at all (very unlikely in my opinion), then all you will have wasted is the current cost of two (or three maximum) cups of coffee in London, or a tiny fraction of the amount of money I and many other people have spent trialling countless ways of trying to beat this very painful and persistent problem.

If this book was available to me at the start of my Plantar Fasciitis journey then it would have saved me thousands of pounds in money, and saved me incredibly painful 24/7 suffering which at times seemed like it would never end.

I hope you find the information in this book of incredible value and I hope that Fix Plantar Fasciitis is the magic, constantly reliable, solution for you that it continues to be for me.

What Are Cheat Sheets?

I have now made Cheat Sheets for you which give you most of the headline points from each section to help easily jog your memory when progressing through your recovery.

There are two separate Cheat Sheets to cover the different stages of recovery and maintenance, and these can be found towards the end of the book.

Structure And Layout Of The Book

I have condensed the information into the shortest notes I could possibly do so that the information is quick to read and easily accessible.

There is a lot of information in this short book but believe me this is a tiny fraction of the information you will encounter in the world out there. However, please don't mistake the information in this book as being limited or incomplete because of the book's short length. The book is deliberately short because it contains the very best information with no fluff or unnecessary content.

The purpose of this short book is to save you time and to give you the best chance of the quickest and most painless recovery.

There are two main sections in the Fix Plantar Fasciitis recovery and prevention book. These represent the stages you may be in your journey to recovery and beyond.

The two main sections are:

Severe Plantar Fasciitis Pain & Beyond

Moderate to Mild Plantar Fasciitis Pain & Beyond

Because the book is aimed to get things fixed as quickly and as easily as possible, it is structured in the order of priority I used, use, and will continue to use in the future if Plantar Fasciitis ever comes back into my life.

I believe the order in which I have presented the information will suit most people.

However, what I suggest is you read through the section which applies to you, and then make your own judgement as to the order and priority which suits you best.

What Are Top Secret Tips

I have highlighted my Top Secret Tips which you may not find that easily elsewhere, but which are my personal top tips for a speedy recovery and healthy foot maintenance.

Some of the tips I give are things which can often be overlooked in favour of the more easily found, run-of-the-mill answers you will find elsewhere.

Some of my tips may be seen as trivial, or minor by people who haven't experienced severe Plantar Fasciitis pain; maybe because the tips can require less effort and/or time to complete than the usual tips you will find. But the tips I give have proven to me that they give a lot more back than you would expect for the amount of effort, and the time they take. Don't dismiss them as trivial or minor, because they have proven to me that they are surprisingly strong.

I don't think you'll find these tips all together in any other book or literature at this point in time, although they are so useful that I do think people will copy me at some point!

What is Plantar Fasciitis?

There is no way I am going to answer this question!

The reason I will not answer this is because you MUST get a diagnosis from your doctor or other suitably qualified medical professional before you can say whether you have Plantar Fasciitis or not, and most definitely before you follow any of the recommendations in this recovery and prevention book.

If you don't know what it is by now, but you do want to know, then you need to search it up and go to the doctor for the diagnosis.

But if you've bought this book then hopefully you know what Plantar Fasciitis is already, you've had a proper diagnosis by a suitable medical professional and are serious about fixing your Plantar Fasciitis as quickly and easily as possible.

Severe Plantar Fasciitis Pain & Beyond

Sleeping

When you sleep you may find that your foot tends to point downwards when resting. This shortens the muscle under your foot and may feel comfortable but will hinder your progress to recovery.

This is because when you get up in the morning your body will have started to heal your Plantar Fasciitis in the shortened position and you will rip this healing progress as soon as you straighten the foot and start walking; hence even more pain.

So, if you do find that your foot wants to naturally point down when resting and sleeping, try to be aware of this and raise your toes and foot to the position it would be in when flat on the floor or when walking. Then the body will begin healing in the lengthened muscle position which is what you want. Some people use a splint to help them achieve this position, but for me it was too painful and uncomfortable to wear at this point in my recovery.

Keep Properly Hydrated

The amount of water recommended for a person to consume per day seems to change all the time, so you need to decide yourself who to listen to regarding this. Your doctor or another health professional you trust can help you.

I can't recommend a specific amount, but my Urologist says to me that when I pee it should look like lemonade, not Lucozade; so I use that as my guide.

Eat A Proper Balanced Diet

Consult your doctor for any special dietary needs or *Do's and Don'ts* in your particular case.

Diet is so important for so many things, it is the basis of your recovery.

I made sure I was getting all of my macros (carbohydrates, proteins, fats), but concentrated on eating lots of fruit, vegetables, and protein for building muscle.

I also supplemented my diet with Vitamin C and Zinc, Vitamin D, and Magnesium (which is also alleged to help you sleep more easily so aiding your recovery even more), but you must check with your doctor before taking any supplements.

Keep Your Muscles Warm And Supple With Good Blood Flow

Your foot, ankle, hip, leg, and back are the first port of call, but the better your entire body is working and the more relaxed and supple it is, then the better your foot will feel and the quicker it will heal. Nothing should be tight (see below for what I do to help stretch and strengthen myself).

Be Like A Child

Be like a child, new to the world with instinctive ways of getting better; don't overthink things.

Think like when you were a child, from that point of view, so you don't let a pain in one part of your body consume you.

Remember how it felt to fall over and graze your knee as a child, and remember how quickly you were able to get over that pain by realising that it was only your knee which was damaged. The rest of your body was not involved with the injury, and you were able to move on with the day very shortly and happily play with your friends again.

As an adult it can be hard to think like this, but you can do it. You've done it before many, many times!

Take Time For Yourself

You are important. You deserve to be loved. You deserve to love yourself.

There is nothing wrong with loving yourself. It doesn't make you arrogant or stand out in a bad way from the crowd. It is good for you to show compassion and caring for yourself.

Spend some time (maybe at the end of the day) slowly feeling the outside of your body, arms, legs, feet etc. with your hands. The purpose is to remind you as an adult that you and your body exist as one. In some cases, to remind yourself that you even have a real body aside from the image you see in the mirror.

With all the distractions of the modern world, with work and family commitments, and with your compassion and caring for others, it is all too easy to let your mind forget about yourself and your body being as one, and being very important.

So, again think like when you were a young child when you were not aware of what may or may not be going on inside your body with the muscles, organs etc. All you knew was the outside and you didn't even think of what was happening on the inside.

You should know now that you will be ok, just like you knew then.

Meditate If You Can

Not all people like the idea of meditation, but my experience with Plantar Fasciitis and also with terrible back problems makes me a big fan of it.

I prefer to do it lying down and I am told that if you are doing a guided meditation (with a spoken voice guiding you), then it doesn't matter if you doze off to sleep at any point as your ears are still listening. I recommend guided meditation.

Take a look at the resource list on the Fix Plantar Fasciitis website (FixPlantarFasciitis.com) to see which meditation resources I have used to help me with severe pain. I have also found the app named Insight Timer to be a very good resource.

Reduce Stress

Yes, this can be much easier said than done; believe me I know. But if I could change one thing in my own life which I knew would help with my health and help with so much more, then it would be to reduce stress. It really does help your body to recover and stay healthy; there is no doubt about that (ask your doctor).

I'm sure you can find many, many resources online and elsewhere to help with your stress. I have put a few items in the Resource List (on FixPlantarFasciitis.com) which I hope will help you like they have helped me.

Meditation and the other tips in this Fix Plantar Fasciitis book will help you to reduce stress; I absolutely believe that. Taking positive steps, with a caring-for-yourself approach towards recovery and maintenance of your health definitely helps you to feel less stressed.

Mobilise Your Ankle And Foot Before Getting Out Of Bed

Yes, it is super tempting to skip this part as it feels pointless when you are in so much pain the moment you get out of bed anyway. But you do really need to do this, and it is easier to quickly do it in bed than in the middle of the day.

What I do is rotate my foot clockwise five times, anticlockwise five times, point my toes five times, and lift my toes towards my shin five times. There are more lengthy alternatives, but I've found that this amount seems to do just well for me.

Avoid Walking With No Shoes On Wooden Or Hard Floors

I'm sure you try to avoid doing this if you have severe pain but make it a priority until the pain is gone. And even after then, my advice is to avoid walking on them too regularly.

Avoid Walking With No Shoes On Cold Floors

Cold may reduce inflammation, so it may be tempting to try to walk on a cold floor, but cold also tends to make your muscles tighten up and shorten, which when combined with walking can make your Plantar Fasciitis worse. If you want to use cold to relieve your pain (usually with an ice pack or similar), then do it whilst sitting or lying down and ask your doctor what she/he recommends regarding the frequency and timings. Too much is too much and too little is too little; ask the professional.

Stairs – Top Secret Tip

When your pain is severe you want to gently stretch the muscles in your foot, but you do not want to force them too hard to stretch (see other exercises and tips below) as this will make your pain even worse.

Walking up the stairs, and down the stairs, puts a lot of stress on the foot and can hinder healing and recovery.

So, to minimise the stress and speed up the recovery I suggest you walk up and down the stairs in a particular way as follows . . .

Walk up and down the stairs one stair at a time with both feet meeting on that stair.

When going up the stairs lead with your good foot (the one without Plantar Fasciitis), follow to the same stair with your bad foot (the one with Plantar Fasciitis), and repeat.

When going down the stairs lead with your bad foot (the one with Plantar Fasciitis), follow to the same stair with your good foot (the one without Plantar Fasciitis), and repeat.

(This tip comes from a surgical expert based in London, UK, who I have full confidence in, but as with all content here you should rely upon your own medical professional for guidance.)

You Need To Have Soft Comfortable Shoes To Relieve The Worst Of The Pain

You need them particularly in the morning when getting out of bed, which can be the most excruciating experience.

The shoes I have found best for this are Crocs (the classic clog shape with the strap at the back to hold them on to your feet).

If you need to go outside for short periods and don't want to wear Crocs then other shoes I have seen recommended include Hoka, Fit Flop, Vionic and many more. However, I can only recommend the ones which worked for me, which remain to this day as Crocs. I believe them to be the best option and it also helps that they are so very easily available.

Do Not Wear Soft Shoes Like Crocs All Day Every Day

Yes, I love them, and I think you will too, and it is very, very tempting to wear the comfortable shoes of your choice all day long. However, in my experience it is all too very easy to get into the mindset of "Well I have no pain, so my Plantar Fasciitis must be getting better!".

Yes, they are helping you to recover, but in my opinion, you must also be restoring the natural strength in your foot (or feet) throughout the whole recovery journey.

Sitting around all day with a trip in your soft shoes to the bathroom and kitchen as your only exercise will only keep you stuck in the 'comfort - zone' and severely slow down your progress to a full recovery.

Do Not Wear Backless Flip-Flops/Thongs Or High Heels At All

It is said that these can shorten your calf muscle, your achilles, and may even have caused your Plantar Fasciitis to occur in the first place.

If you choose to wear the Crocs without the heel strap, then make sure you are not 'holding' them on (with your toes when you lift your feet to walk) in the same way you would hold Flip-Flops/Thongs on. It's a natural and subtle movement, but it's more than enough to make your Plantar Fasciitis worse, and to eve bring it back after having recovered.

High heeled shoes have the added problem that they tend to be pointed at the front and restrict the movement of your toes, and the blood flow, (see below for more info on this). Don't wear them.

Do not shorten your calf muscle and achilles tendon. You need to have your body working as it would naturally before Flip-Flops and High Heels were invented!

Do Not Sit Down All Day

You need to get your feet and legs moving.

Sitting reduces, and can in some cases restrict, the blood flow to your legs and feet.

You need to be strengthening yourself from day one, so move about but be gentle on yourself.

Don't try to do too much at first but do make a note of how much movement you are doing. Yes, it can seem a bit of a bind to make a note every time you move, but if you can make a quick note when you do (it doesn't have to be noted 'to the second'!), then you will be able to track your progress and feel better quicker. Having done this I know how much such a simple thing can help.

When Sitting On A High Dining Chair Or Office Chair –
Top Secret Tip

Some people when sitting on a higher chair have a tendency to point one toe resting on the ground under the chair and then rest the other leg on the achilles of the leg with the pointed toe. Do not do this even though it feels comfortable as it has hindered my progress and I think will most likely hinder yours too.

Clothing

Do not wear restrictive clothing.

What I mean by this in particular is do not wear socks or anything else which restricts your blood flow. For example do not wear trousers which reduce your blood flow or pull on your body, back, legs, or anywhere when you move or are sitting down. However subtle or small the tightening, pulling, and restriction may feel on your body, it can have a big negative effect on your recovery.

I have found the 'pulling' has the largest negative effect and has been a part of clothing for so many of us for so long that we don't even take much or any notice of it. For instance, tight trousers or jeans which have a low waist seem to be a real villain.

When you think about it, tight clothing pulling on your body, particularly from the waist down, is directly affecting the fascia by adding another (alien) layer to your body which is in the 'wrong' place (i.e. directly outside your skin) and is in effect replacing some of the job of your muscles and fascia itself. Again, this might seem very minor, and you might want to skip this point, but it really does affect the body.

Tight, pulling clothes are something to bin, and personally I will never take the risk of going back to them.

You need to wear warm, good fitting clothing, which is comfortable and does not restrict your movement, but which you don't feel is too loose to the point that you are holding yourself in a strange way to hold things in the right place (however minor it may seem; you may not even have noticed you are doing it until you turn your conscious attention to it).

You will find throughout this book that subtlety in many things all can have a massive effect on your recovery.

Footwear In General And Social Media

Understandably, there is a LOT of discussion about footwear and Plantar Fasciitis. You will find this particularly on Facebook groups and other social media. Believe me, I've been there.

Personally, I think that these places can make things even more confusing, and I also think that the advice you find and may take literally depends on the day or short period you visit and it may not be the best advice at all.

A lot of people seem to get stuck on those groups in the severe phase and don't seem to recover very quickly, if at all.

I found that there is a lot of comfort advice. A lot of "which shoes are the most comfortable?" advice. This is because understandably most people are in the severe phase when they reach out for help, so all they want and need at that point is quick relief from the terrible pain. Crocs and similar footwear (see the Resource List on FixPlantarFasciitis.com) provide this quick relief, but I don't think they alone can make you recover unless your pain is not actually as severe as it can be. What I mean by this is that you may not be anywhere near the pinnacle of Plantar pain even though you think you are. I've had many injuries and other pains during my life so far and Plantar Fasciitis at its most severe is high up on the list.

With footwear, the hard truth of the matter is that you will find you are juggling a lot of different shoes during your recovery and beyond.

That is what you must do to maximise your chances of recovery, to minimise the time it takes, and to maintain your foot strength and mobility so as to help prevent any recurrence.

You will also find that you use certain shoes to help stop, or to quickly and immediately stop, a suspected recurrence.

What shoes work for one person may not work for you. And you will find that nothing makes sense at all at times; until you start to work things out through trial and error. You will get there sooner than you may think, and you will probably find that you have a very small stock of shoes which you know to wear for different situations and self-therapy.

However, I am here to guide you in this book as to what I recommend from my research (including hours and hours on Facebook groups) and my pain, and I'm here to give you some good pointers which I believe will help you with your footwear to minimise your pain and maximise the speed of your recovery.

Existing Footwear

Make sure your existing shoes aren't worn down or misshapen because you need to get your feet to behave as they would be doing naturally when you were a child.

Existing shoes could be shaped to the way you have been walking with Plantar Fasciitis if you have had them a long time. And existing shoes could have caused the Plantar Fasciitis or contributed to it.

This applies to the uppers, and the heel and soles; to every part of the shoe!

New Footwear

If you can get some new shoes, then do.

Make sure you get shoes which fit your foot well, are supportive, but not restrictive, and which have good arch support.

I recommend you get shoes with laces so you can adjust the tension and fit to be most comfortable.

Make sure you have a lot of room in the new shoes for your toes to spread at the front of the shoe. People talk of shoes known specifically as 'wide toe box' shoes, which I do recommend (I use some wide toe-box shoes made by Altra), but you can find other shoes which have a wider toe area than normal, and I have a great Top Secret Tip about how to help spread your toes in lace up shoes below for you too.

If you can have gait analysis (see below) and get advice on new shoes specific to your gait from an expert, then definitely take the opportunity to do so when you are ready.

Tight Fitting Shoes

The temptation may be to buy tight fitting shoes. These can appear to give instant relief, and they can, but in reality this tends to be very short lived. A tight pair of shoes can actually hinder the strengthening of your foot and it's recovery if worn for long periods of time without swapping with other types of shoe.

There are differences between tight and well fitted. You want well fitted.

I must admit that I fell for the super-supportive shoe idea and bought some. I did feel instant relief, which could even last for a few hours. But it definitely stalled my recovery, and may have made things worse.

In conjunction with the advice I am providing in this book, it wasn't until I used a combination of well- fitted, supportive shoes, Crocs, and wide toe box shoes (in my case Altra) that I fully recovered and was able to properly gain and maintain strength in my feet.

Conversely (no shoe pun intended), someone very close to me who had similar foot problems to myself (although no way near as severe), wore their super-supportive (over-supportive) shoes, still does today, and they still have pain.

You need to have good blood flow to, around, and from your feet. Over supportive shoes can restrict this if you are not careful.

You need to be strengthening your feet. Over supportive shoes can hinder this strengthening by doing too much 'work' for you.

For me, after much trial and error, the 'perfect' supportive shoe ended up being the Merrell Moab 3, but for you it may be something different, although Merrell made shoes come highly recommended by many Plantar Fasciitis sufferers.

Get the advice of an expert, try on as many different shoes as you can until they fit you like a comfortable, supportive, warm (but not hot) glove.

Also check out the list of shoes I have seen repeatedly recommended in Facebook groups and elsewhere when I was searching for the perfect pair. You can find this list in the Resource List on the Fix Plantar Fasciitis website (FixPlantarFasciitis.com).

Insoles (A.K.A. Innersoles)

If you have good shoes already, or even if you buy new ones and find they aren't quite doing the job, it may be worth investing in some insoles.

I have tried a lot of different insoles and spent a fortune doing so. Hopefully, you won't have to as there are two which I have bought more than once to aid my recovery.

The first one which I recommend for starting your journey when your pain is severe to moderate are . . .

FootActive COMFORT Premium Insoles

. . . because they are softer than some and have a very good heel cushion which can really help to ease the pain. So, if that particular brand and model are not available where you are then look for those attributes.

The second set I recommend for being supportive, relatively cheap, and good quality, but more suited to when your pain is less severe are . . .

PRO 11 WELLBEING Plantar Series Orthotic Insoles

. . . which I have repeat purchased many times for many shoes, and will continue to wear.

Don't expect insoles to take your pain completely away when you are at the severe stage. They don't in my experience, but they do make it easier, which helps you to start moving more and can aid your recovery.

Roomy Toes And A Whole Lot More – A Top Secret Top 3 Tip

This is one of the best tips I can give you.

It is one which I use every single day, and most importantly it is one which gives a massive amount of benefit with very little effort.

It's quick, easy, and still gives me surprisingly great results. Plus, it only takes a few seconds to do. This is it:

When you are putting your shoes on do this . . .

1. Sit down.
2. Loosen your laces and put your foot into your shoe.
3. With the laces loosened, and your foot flat in the shoe, curl your toes downwards and under (as if to make a fist with them).
4. Do not force your toes to make a tense fist, just curl them without straining.
5. Whilst in this position, gently but firmly (not tightly) secure the laces starting at the toe end and working up to the ankle until you have tied the bow.
6. Release the curled toes.
7. Repeat with the other foot and shoe.
8. Walk, and thank me later! You will be amazed at how comfortable but supportive your shoes feel, but more to the point this allows better toe spread and better blood flow to your feet, and you know how important that is to healing your Plantar Fasciitis.

Toe Socks

I'm a big fan of toe separating socks and strongly believe they helped my recovery.

At first they felt uncomfortable, and I found them hard to get on my feet. This is normal for most people.

But once you get used to them, they're brilliant as they let your foot behave more naturally, as it was designed to do. They definitely help with strengthening your foot.

The toe socks I have are from Amazon and are from the more budget friendly brands and they suit my needs just fine.

Allegedly Injinji toe socks are the most well-established brand and seen as the best but are more expensive.

Toe Separators/Toe Spreaders

Another brilliant tool to use to regain your natural foot shape.

Do check with your medical professional to see that they are suitable for you if you have any doubts, but what I did was buy some and I wore them for short periods of time around the house. They are too uncomfortable for me to wear in my shoes outside the house.

The toe separators I bought and used are silicone, as I can't imagine using the harder ones that are also available. These are the ones I bought . . .

YogaMedic® Toe Separator for Overlapping Toes 4Pcs Improved Silicone, 0% BPA

. . . but I'm sure they don't have to be brand specific.

Walk

Yes, it sounds like the worst thing to do because, it can be utterly unbearable with the pain; believe me I know. But you must mobilise your foot, ankle, leg, and body.

You must try to move as naturally and without stiffness as much as possible.

Try (it can be hard) to relax and to take it slowly at first and walk in your home with your soft shoes.

Progress to walking longer (but still short) distances in the correct shoes as soon as you can.

Stretch

You must have good mobility in your body, but aside from the feet and ankles, particularly the next areas in the kinetic chain which are your legs and back.

There are so many stretch videos and stretch instructions available within easy reach today that you really need to find what personally suits you best. You also need to consult your chosen medical professional before doing any stretches.

But, as you know by now, I have tried loads (over many years) until I found the most effective and least time-consuming stretches which work for me. So, I can give you this information here and hopefully you'll find these stretches as beneficial as I do.

When you do any stretches, never force them. Treat yourself as if you are gently helping your most precious person who you love the most in the world. You need to love yourself like this.

It took many years for both myself and friends who have had injuries, sports injuries and pain related to age and illness to realise that stretching really does need to be gentle to be most effective. Straining, particularly in the early stages of recovery is not the way to stretch.

Epsom Salts

I recommend using Epsom Bath Salts in a large bowl big enough to accommodate your feet if you are ok to without any adverse reaction.

I recommend doing this as often as you can safely do (check with your chemist/pharmacist and/or your medical professional).

This is again another thing which people see as minor, and not worth the effort, but which can really help.

Tiger Balm

Something which can sometimes be seen as 'not scientifically proven' by the naysayers, I actually had great results using Tiger Balm on the underside of my feet. Better than any other of the skin applied ointments or creams, including the medicated ones. I don't know why, but Tiger Balm just seems to work to lower the pain and aid heeling. Always check with your health professional if you are ok to use this.

How I Stretch My Back And The Backs Of My Legs – Top Secret Tip

When it comes to stretching my back and legs, there is one simple exercise which I always use. This is how I do it:

1. Stand up straight with feet together.
2. Keeping your heels together rotate your toes away from each other, pivoting on your heels, so that your feet are now 45 degrees diagonal to your body, forming a V shape when you look down.
3. Put your toes back onto the floor and then pivot on them, moving your heels now so that your feet are parallel again but approximately now shoulder width apart.
4. Now relax and bend forward at the hip as if to touch your toes, with your arms and fingers hanging down.
5. You MUST NOT push or force your body to try to stretch. This is very important, as I have found to my detriment on a few occasions when I have been in a hurry for whatever reason and have thought I would be ok to push a little. Do not.
6. Now take a deep breath. But visualize that you are actually taking the breath deep into your lower back. Breathe out slowly, and repeat. Relax more with each breath. Let your own weight do the work, not your muscles.

7. Once you feel you have relaxed enough throughout the length of your stretch, then slowly and carefully straighten yourself to a full standing position.

When done correctly you will be amazed at how much your body will relax and how much lower down your hands will go. I have on many an occasion started the stretch, and my fingertips are 12 inches or more away from my toes. And by the end of the stretch (I may have to repeat it twice) my fingers invariably reach my toes without me having to push or force anything at all. But, like I say, do not force it; the object of the exercise is to release tension and to allow your body to stretch, not to reach your toes.

It is all done with relaxation allowing your body to free itself from tension naturally.

How I Stretch The Front Of My Thigh

1. Standing straight, with your feet together or slightly apart.
2. You will be standing on one leg in the next step, so make sure you can either do this ok already or position yourself with something firm enough to hold on to if you need to help yourself balance.
3. Now lift one foot off the floor and backwards, bending at the knee. Again, you must make sure you are physically ok to do any of these stretches prior to doing them (check with your doctor if not sure).
4. Next grab the lifted foot behind you and pull gently towards your back.
5. Relax into it.
6. Breathe into it.
7. Hold for up to 30 seconds, but any time is fine if it suits you; do not strain.
8. Slowly release and steadily place your foot back on the floor.
9. Repeat the procedure with the other leg.

10. Repeat three times, or whatever feels most comfortable for you, but as with all stretches, don't do too many the first few times, 'just because you can', because you may regret it later.

IMHO The Best Local Stretch For Plantar Fasciitis – Top Secret Top 3 Tip

This stretch appears to be the opposite of what most Plantar Fasciitis remedies tell you. But in my experience it is stretch which can produce magical relief and healing results. It is also a stretch which I now use to curtail any suspected recurrence of Plantar Fasciitis at the first signs. Here it is . . .

When sitting, do the following, preferably on a carpet, rug, cushion or deep pillow if easier (usually if you are very tight or at the beginning of your recovery):

1. On your (bare or socked) foot with Plantar Fasciitis, curl your toes under.
2. Lift your foot off the ground (or cushion), heel up, toes down.
3. Point your foot down and rest your curled toes on the floor or cushion, or something soft but not slippery.
4. Gently stretch the top of your foot by gently pushing down and forward.
5. Hold for five or more seconds, but don't rush. If you want to gently hold for slightly longer then that is fine. Do what gets the best results for you.
6. Repeat three to five times.
7. Do this stretch three times per day or whatever you find suits you the best.

Stretches For Strengthening Whilst Sitting Day-To-Day

When sitting, I also do the following two exercises:

1. Feet flat on the floor, curl your toes under, hold for a count of five, release. Repeat five times, or whatever is comfortable for you.

2. Feet flat on the floor, lift your toes up (using your muscles only), hold for the count of five, release. Repeat five times, or whatever is comfortable for you.

I recommend doing these throughout the day, whenever you are sitting down (remember not to sit down for the whole day). The maximum I would do these is five times per day; but experiment and do whatever suits you.

You will probably see many people recommending to do the second stretch (toes up) by pulling with your hands on the foot/toes. I tried this, and it made things worse.

I think pulling with the hands can tempt people to pull too hard and rip the injury to the fascia way too much.

So, in my opinion, you should not do the one where you are pulling with your hands because you will get enough mobility from doing it with your muscles only and then when you walk, your foot will be more able to stretch any extra distance it needs, which will further help your return to natural, unhindered, movement.

Ball And / Or Roller Under The Foot

You will see people recommending rollers and balls for rolling under your feet when you are sitting down. I too recommend them, but as with everything here, do small amounts, gently and often as opposed to going full throttle at it thinking you will get a speedier recovery. Your recovery will be faster if you do small amounts, gently and often.

The best items I have used, and continue to use, for rolling under your feet (again after much trial and error) are:

These balls: Beenax Lacrosse & Hard Spiky Massage Ball Set

This roller: Due North Foot Rubz Foot Massage Roller

I don't think you have to be too specific about the makes and manufacturers as long as the items are good quality.

I find the smoothness of the Lacrosse Ball gently lengthens and loosens the muscle, tendons and fascia, whereas the hard spiky options seem to increase the blood flow and stimulation to the area, which in my opinion helps the body to repair and heal.

As with all recommendations in this book, including exercises, use these mindfully, gently thinking about what you are doing and how your body is healing as you use the exercises and items.

Calf Roller

For me the use of a calf roller really helped.

If you imagine the muscles and tendons being tight down the back of your leg, around the back of your heel, under your foot, and in to your toes, then you can imagine that making sure this whole area is supple and healthy can play a big part in helping your plantar fasciitis.

The roller I use is listed below, but I have seen people using wooden rolling pins (and other devices) and if my plastic roller ever breaks, then I will definitely try a rolling pin to see how that fairs.

This is the roller I use: Physix Muscle Roller Stick

You can also, like me, use the roller on your shin muscle (not bone), and upper leg muscles too to help keep things supple and with good blood flow. It's definitely worth having.

Gait And Kinetic Chain

You will normally find that the foot which has the Plantar Fasciitis and/or that side of your body has something odd about the way it behaves and moves. I believe this can be the cause of the Plantar Fasciitis.

It may have been brought about by an injury and not noticed for years, but it can be caused by anything in the kinetic chain from the tips of your toes right the way up your entire body to the top of your head.

It can also be caused by something in the other foot or the other side of your body.

If you can find where you are moving in a different way than you would expect from a brand new, fully healthy body, then you may well have discovered the source of the problem or a contributary factor.

For me I eventually discovered that a contributary factor in my Plantar Fasciitis started in my back, then to abdomen, and finally into the foot.

And if you're like me then you may discover that the source of at least some of your problem is similar.

Your body really is one unit and relies on all the parts working the best they can.

When you walk, from this point in time onwards, be consciously aware of:

1. Your Gait
   Are you walking as you would have done when you were 'brand new'? Your kinetic chain from your toes to your head should be properly aligned and walking with relaxed confidence.
2. Your Foot Position And How You Place Your feet When you Are Walking – Top Secret Tip
   Is one foot placement and position different from the other? Could you demonstrate the 'perfect' walk to another person learning to walk?
3. Foot Drop Or Slanting
   Is there any foot drop or slanting/angling of the foot when you walk? This could be either when you lift the foot, when you place the foot to the ground, or both.

Replicate – Top Secret Tip

When looking at your body and kinetic chain in the points above, do you have one side of your body which you feel is normal (or 'more normal') than the other side? If you do, then try to replicate the way that side moves and behaves on the other side.

Dominant Side – Top Secret Top 3 Tip

If I was forced to choose one Top Secret Tip from them all then this one would be right up there at the top very closely followed by my Top 3 Tips named 'Local Stretch' and 'Roomy Toes'. Here it is . . .

When walking, you will most likely find that one foot, ankle, leg, and/or hip is dominant over the other.

This can present itself in many different ways, but it is likely you will find that you are propelling your body forward more strongly from one side than the other.

Obviously, when you are in severe pain then that will be because of your pain in your foot, making the other one work harder.

But, and this is the crux of it, when you have recovered and have no pain you will probably find that you still have a dominant side; and you most likely did before the pain began.

You need to be balanced on both sides, so begin now.

What you need to do is:

1. Be aware of your dominant side.
2. Make a mental note whilst walking of how your dominant side, particularly your leg, hip and foot, are moving and behaving. Where is the power coming from? How does the leg and foot behave? How is everything aligned?
3. Mentally switch your dominant side to your other side. Make this the current dominant side and replicate how your original dominant side was behaving. Concentrate on every part of your stepping motion.
4. Concentrate on being comfortable using this new side as your current dominant side, but don't strain or tense up to try to

progress faster, because this will hinder your progress and may even cause your pain to get worse.

5. At first just do this for a short distance, maximum twenty steps.

6. Repeat the process of studying your naturally dominant leg and foot behaviour.

7. Switch back to replicating the dominant behaviour on your non-dominant side.

8. Do this during your recovery, lengthening the time and walking distance you swap the dominant behaviour to your non-dominant side.

9. Monitor your progress carefully. If you feel like you have made your pain worse or caused any other discomfort which you think could become persistent, then reduce back to less time and distance until your body heals and catches up. It may seem like a delay, but in reality, it may only take a few days or a week for your body to heal and allow you to progress again.

10. Continue doing this forever! Yes, I know you were probably hoping that once it's done, it's done, but I have found in my experience that the body naturally wants to go back to 'comfortable' and dare I say 'lazy' habits, and this 'natural' relaxation of a non-dominant side is one of them. So, monitor how you are stepping every time you walk. This is very important to your recovery and maintenance.

Moderate To Mild Plantar Fasciitis Pain & Beyond

Continue with any or all of the tips in the Severe Plantar Fasciitis Pain section when your pain is moderate or mild. This is with a view to gradually dropping the ones which you don't feel you need anymore as your recovery progresses. But you may find that some stick with you right through your entire recovery and even into the rest of your life, so you can live it to the fullest.

Get Gait Analysis And Video Yourself Walking

If you have somewhere (like a running shop) where you can go to get your gait analysed, then I recommend you do this.

Check before you go if they are set up to do walking only gait analysis if you are still unable to run.

They will be able to give you an amazing amount of information about how you are moving, how to remedy certain issues in your movement, and also they will be able to recommend footwear specifically for you.

You need to tell them about your Plantar Fasciitis and any other issues you have, and they will usually perform a questionnaire on you before doing the analysis.

Whether you are able or unable to get gait analysis, I also recommend that you video yourself walking. Get someone to do it from a short distance, from both sides, and from front and back. Do it for a good number of steps outside where you would normally walk; and just walk as you would day to day.

Once you have done this, then ask someone to video you walking more closely with the camera pointing towards your feet.

Yes, you are probably not an expert, but you will be amazed at what you can see in the videos of you moving.

Looking closely, you will see that you are most likely not moving in exactly the way you thought.

There will be discrepancies between one side of your body and the other.

You will see how you are lifting your feet, how you are placing your feet, and how you are propelling your body when walking.

This will allow you to work towards making your movements balanced on both sides, which is vital for a healthy recovery and strong maintenance.

Stairs When Pain Is Reducing

When your pain is reduced it is important that you walk up stairs as you would have done before the pain started.

You need to get mobile and strong in the areas which Plantar Fasciitis has stolen from you.

But take it easy at first. Do not run up or down the stairs. Walk with confidence and gentle purpose, monitoring your foot placement and movement.

This is one time where I recommend that you let your naturally dominant foot (without Plantar Fasciitis) be the leader for a while until you are feeling like your non-dominant foot is as strong as your dominant foot.

By doing the exercises I have suggested, and by walking according to the dominant side technique I have explained at length in this book, you should soon find that your non-dominant foot gains the strength and mobility you need to walk up and down stairs again normally.

Shoes

When you're ready, you may like to try zero-drop shoes. I don't recommend you try barefoot shoes at this stage but get some zero-drop shoes which have some padding.

Altra are my chosen brand for this (having researched extensively, and subsequently wearing them regularly).

You will need to double check you are actually buying shoes which are zero-drop, and I definitely recommend that you choose a shoe with a wide toe box so you can let your feet work as they are designed to do, not necessarily how we have been told by the big brands.

When you are better, if you find you want to try barefoot shoes, proceed cautiously and research what you need to do to ease into wearing them. Vivobarefoot are one of the most well-known barefoot shoe companies, but there are many other brands available now.

Walk More

Walk often and for longer distances. For me that meant walking one mile per day, then progressing to two miles per day (one mile in one direction, and after a rest or later in the day, one mile back) as I got better and stronger.

Stretches And Strength Training

Walking correctly, with the 'dominant side', foot positioning and your gait in mind always, in my opinion is the best natural strengthening you can do.

Also continue to do the stretches and strength exercises I have outlined. You must keep your legs and feet soft and supple, and may also want to employ the help of a massage therapist if this helps you to do this.

Have Baths

If you have severe pain, then I do recommend this too. However, at one point due to the severity of the pain I couldn't even face the idea of stepping in to and out of a bath tub.

But when you can, I think you should.

Baths seem to get a bad rap these days in favour of showers, but I believe in the power of the bath. Not only does it relax you, it hydrates your skin for far longer than a quick shower.

And I recommend using Epsom Bath Salts in your bath if you are ok to do that without any adverse reaction. They definitely seem to help even more with relaxation and with Plantar Fasciitis. I do this once per week.

Sleep More

I'm sure you realise the importance of good sleep.

Unfortunately, I know that sleep can scare you when you have severe Plantar Fasciitis pain as you dread the prospect of getting up in the morning and the pain potentially (likely) being even worse because of a longer sleep with your foot in the 'wrong' position (see Sleep section above).

But hopefully now you are able to sleep better with less pain, and with less dread of the morning, so take advantage of that.

Make sure you get good lengths of sleep.

Plus, I find that if I let myself sleep in for longer on Sunday, for instance, then my whole body feels like it's heeled itself much more than the shorter sleeps during the rest of the week. Even though I try to get good length of sleep on those days too, in reality I rarely do. A long sleep at least once per week definitely seems to help.

When You Are Almost Plantar Fasciitis Pain Free:

- Walk barefoot at home if possible, at least for a few trips around the house.
- If you feel pain then don't do it; stop it completely until you can do it without any pain at all.
- Make more walks up stairs. If painful then take it slowly but do do it.
- Again, concentrate on your foot positioning being normal. Don't compensate for the pain unless absolutely necessary, and reduce the amount of times you are training on the stairs.
- Mix your footwear between Crocs, normal shoes, and Altras/zero-drop wide toebox shoes (or if very strong then add barefoot shoes too).
- Use these in balance to suit your needs, so if you feel some pain coming back, then move the balance from Altra/zero-drop to Crocs, with normal shoes as the pivot point of the scale.
- Continue to always monitor your gait, dominant side, dominant foot, foot positioning, foot angle, and check if you are dragging a foot.
- Walk with confidence and purpose, but not so that you are over emphasising any movements.
- Be gentle on yourself remembering that your feet are part of you even if they are painful, and they are not the enemy.
- **Know for sure that you will be strong and you will fix your Plantar Fasciitis.**

TERMS & CONDITIONS

These Terms and Conditions apply to all areas of the Fix Plantar Fasciitis Book, FixPlantarFasciitis.com, and any other related material.

I do not possess medical qualifications or expertise. Attempting any remedies or techniques described carries inherent risks. Proceed with caution, using sound judgment, and immediately cease any activities causing pain or discomfort. The information provided serves informational purposes only.

The content available, encompassing written material, visuals, and data, does not substitute professional medical counsel, diagnosis or treatment plans. It presents general knowledge that may change without prior notification. Confirm any information from additional sources and review all health-related matters with licensed medical practitioners.

Under no circumstances should you disregard professional medical advice or postpone seeking treatment based solely on the content accessible through this platform.

No endorsements or claims are made regarding the efficacy, suitability or appropriateness of any specific tests, products, procedures, treatments, services, opinions, healthcare providers or other information that may be present.

We hold no responsibility or liability for any guidance, course of action, diagnosis or other information, services, or products you may obtain through accessing this content.

The information provided in this book is based on personal experience and research and should not be construed as professional medical advice. Readers are encouraged to consult with a qualified healthcare professional for individualized medical guidance.

The information is not intended as a substitute for professional medical advice, diagnosis, or treatment. Always seek the advice of your physician or other qualified healthcare provider with any questions you may have regarding a medical condition.

The author and publisher of this book, the information on FixPlantarFasciitis.com and related material, shall not be liable for any direct, indirect, incidental, special, or consequential damages arising out of or relating to the use of the information provided.

While every effort has been made to ensure the accuracy and reliability of the information presented, the author and publisher make no representations or warranties regarding the completeness, accuracy, suitability, or reliability of the content. The information is provided 'as is' without warranty of any kind, either express or implied.

The experiences and outcomes described in this book are based on the author's personal journey and may not be typical or representative of every reader's experience. Results may vary depending on individual circumstances.

The information is based on the author's personal experiences and is not intended to be a substitute for professional medical advice, diagnosis, or treatment. The views and opinions expressed are solely those of the author and do not necessarily reflect those of any medical professional or organization.

By reading this book, readers acknowledge that they understand and accept the risks associated with implementing any suggestions or recommendations. It is recommended to consult with a healthcare professional before making any changes to medical treatment or lifestyle.

Any disputes arising from the use of this book shall be governed by the laws of England, UK and shall be subject to the exclusive jurisdiction of the courts in England, UK.

The author strongly encourages readers to consult with qualified medical professionals for any medical concerns or conditions they may have. The information provided in this book should not be used as a basis for self-diagnosis or self-treatment.

As eBooks cannot be returned we are unable to refund payments. By completing the purchase of an eBook from FixPlantarFasciitis.com you waive your 14 day right to cancel. If the product is found to be faulty then you can get a refund, but please be aware that all products are tested for faults before sending to the purchaser. This policy does not affect your Statutory Rights.

These Terms and Conditions apply to all areas of FixPlantarFasciitis.com, the Fix Plantar Fasciitis eBook, Book, and to the transactions related to our products and services, and are in conjunction with our full Terms and Conditions on our website FixPlantaarFasciitis.com which you will have agreed to by checkbox consent prior to purchasing the eBook. You may be bound by additional contracts related to your relationship with us or any products or services that you receive from us. If any provisions of the additional contracts conflict with any provisions of these Terms, the provisions of these additional contracts will control and prevail.

Severe Pain – Cheat Sheet

It is important to use the full instructions in the Fix Plantar Fasciitis book, but this cheat sheet will help you to jog your memory of some of the tips included.

1. **Sleeping**

   - Avoid pointing your foot downwards when resting or sleeping.
   - Keep your foot in a flat or toe slightly raised position similar to when walking to aid healing.

2. **Hydration**

   - Stay properly hydrated.
   - Aim for urine colour resembling lemonade.

3. **Balanced Diet**

   - Consult a doctor for dietary advice.
   - Focus on fruits, vegetables, and protein.
   - Consider supplements like Vitamin C, Zinc, Vitamin D, and Magnesium after consulting a doctor that these would be suitable for you.

4. **Muscle Warmth And Blood Flow**

   - Maintain good blood flow and muscle suppleness, especially in foot, ankle, leg, hip, and back.

5. **Childlike Attitude**

   - Approach pain with the resilience of a child.
   - Don't let pain consume you; affected areas are the only painful places.

6. **Self-Care**

- Dedicate time for self-love and compassion.
- Connect with your body through gentle touch and acknowledgment.

7. **Meditation**

- Consider meditation to manage pain and stress.

8. **Stress Reduction**

- Reduce stress to aid recovery.
- Utilize meditation and self-care practices.

9. **Mobilize Before Getting Out Of Bed**

- Perform ankle and foot mobilization exercises before getting out of bed.

10. **Avoid Barefoot Walking**

- Avoid and prevent walking barefoot on hard or cold floors, especially with severe pain.

11. **Stair Walking Technique**

- Use our specific stair-walking technique to minimize stress on the foot.

12. **Comfortable Footwear**

- Use soft, comfortable shoes like Crocs, especially in the morning.
- Avoid wearing them all day every day to prevent reliance on comfort.

13. **Avoid Flip-Flops/Thongs And High Heels**

- Steer clear of backless flip-flops/thongs and high heels to prevent further strain on the foot.

14. Avoid Prolonged Sitting

- Ensure regular movement to prevent reduced blood flow and stiffness.

15. Be Aware Of Sitting Habits

- Avoid resting one foot on the achilles of the other leg when sitting.

16. Wear Comfortable Clothing

- Opt for loose, comfortable clothing that promotes warmth and good blood flow.

17. Footwear Selection

- Choose supportive shoes with good arch support and ample toe room.
- Consider lace-up shoes for adjustability.

18. Beware Of Tight Shoes

- Differentiate between tight and well-fitted shoes to avoid hindering foot recovery.

19. Footwear Assessment

- Evaluate existing footwear for wear and tear which can affect recovery.

20. Invest In New Footwear

- Invest in new shoes with good support and proper fit.

21. Insoles (A.K.A. Innersoles)

- Consider using insoles for additional support and comfort.

22. Roomy Toes Technique

- Follow our specific lacing technique to promote toe spread and better blood flow.

23. Toe Socks

- Consider using toe separating socks to aid foot recovery.

24. Toe Separators

- Use toe separators to restore natural foot shape and mobility.

25. Maintain Regular Walking

- Mobilize your foot and leg muscles by walking regularly, starting with short distances.

26. Stretching

- Incorporate gentle stretching exercises for overall body mobility and muscle flexibility.

27. Back And Leg Stretching Technique

- Practice our specific stretching exercise for back and leg flexibility.

28. Thigh Stretching

- Perform gentle thigh stretches to promote flexibility and mobility.

29. Local Stretch For Feet

- Follow our 'secret' stretching exercise targeting the top of the foot.

30. Sitting Stretching Exercises

- Incorporate seated stretching exercises to strengthen foot muscles.

31. Ball And Roller Under Foot

- Use balls and rollers to gently massage and stretch foot muscles; do not push hard or for too long.

32. Calf Roller

- Utilize a calf roller to maintain suppleness and blood flow in the calf muscles.

33. Gait And Kinetic Chain

- Assess your walking pattern and body alignment for potential contributing factors to Plantar Fasciitis.

34. Dominant Side

- Try to replicate the movement and behaviour of your dominant side on the non-dominant side.
- Switch dominant sides to promote balanced movement and prevent strain.

This condensed cheat sheet offers actionable tips with the aim of managing Plantar Fasciitis effectively.

Remember to consult with a medical professional for personalized advice and treatment before actioning any of the tips.

Remember, this is just a Cheat Sheet for quick reference and does not contain all of the tips, or any detail. Full details of the tips are in the book Fix Plantar Fasciitis from FixPlantarFasciitis.com

Moderate To Mild Pain – Cheat Sheet

It is important to use the full instructions in the Fix Plantar Fasciitis book, but this cheat sheet will help you to jog your memory of some of the main tips included.

1. **Gait Analysis And Video Walking**

   - Visit a running shop or similar for gait analysis.
   - Inform them about your condition and any related issues.
   - Video yourself walking from various angles.
   - Analyze your movement for discrepancies and imbalance.
   - Work towards balanced movements for healthy recovery.

2. **Stairs**

   - Gradually reintroduce stair walking as pain reduces.
   - Walk up stairs with confidence and purpose; but do not run.
   - Allow the dominant foot to lead initially.
   - Focus on foot placement and movement.
   - Strengthen non-dominant foot over time.

3. **Shoes**

   - Transition to zero-drop shoes with padding.
   - Choose shoes with a wide toe box for natural foot movement.
   - Consider brands like Altra for zero-drop shoes.
   - Proceed cautiously with barefoot shoes, if you choose to, when ready.

4. **Walk More**

   - Increase walking frequency and distance gradually.
   - Start with one mile per day, progress as strength improves.

5. **Stretches And Strength Training**

- Prioritize correct walking technique and foot positioning.
- Continue recommended stretches and strength exercises.

When Almost Pain Free . . .

1. **Barefoot Walking**

- Walk barefoot (keep feet warm with socks if necessary) at home, for short periods, without pain.
- Stop if pain occurs or increases and resume when pain-free.

2. **Stair Walking**

- Increase frequency of stair walking gradually.
- Maintain normal foot positioning and movement.

3. **Mix Footwear**

- Rotate between Crocs, Normal Shoes, and Altras/zero-drop shoes.
- Adjust balance between shoe types based on pain levels.
- Use footwear to suit comfort and recovery needs.

4. **Monitor Gait**

- Continuously assess gait, foot positioning, and movement.
- Address any abnormalities promptly.

5. **Walk Confidently**

- Walk with confidence and purpose, but not to abnormal levels.
- Avoid overemphasizing movements.

6. **Be Gentle**

- Treat your feet kindly and avoid self-blame.
- Understand that recovery takes time and patience.

7. **Stay Positive**

- Believe in your ability to overcome Plantar Fasciitis.
- Focus on strength and resilience throughout recovery.
- **You can fix your Plantar Fasciitis.**

This condensed cheat sheet offers actionable tips with the aim of managing Plantar Fasciitis effectively. Remember to consult with a medical professional for personalized advice and treatment before actioning any of the tips.

Remember, this is just a Cheat Sheet for quick reference and it doesn't contain all of the tips or the details in the book. Full details of the tips are in the book Fix Plantar Fasciitis from FixPlantarFasciitis.com